Confronting the Big C

A Family Faces Cancer

Confronting the Big C

Henry D. Weaver

with Mary E. Weaver *(Wife)*
Sally Weaver Glick *(Daughter)*
Judy Weaver Aguirre *(Daughter)*
Debora J. Weaver *(Daughter)*
Joseph Donald Weaver *(Son)*

Illustrations by Sallie J. Weaver
(Mother, drawn at age 91)

HERALD PRESS
Scottdale, Pennsylvania
Kitchener, Ontario
1984

Library of Congress Cataloging in Publication Data

Weaver, Henry D., 1928-
  Confronting the big C.

    1. Weaver, Henry D., 1928-   . 2. Cancer—Patients—United
States—Biography. 3. Cancer—Patients—Family relationships.
4. Cancer—Psychological aspects.
I. Title.
RC265.6.W43A34   1984   362.1'96994'00924 [B]   84-15638
ISBN 0-8361-3373-0 (pbk.)

CONFRONTING THE BIG C
Copyright © 1984 by Herald Press, Scottdale, Pa. 15683
    Published simultaneously in Canada by Herald Press,
    Kitchener, Ont. N2G 4M5. All rights reserved.
Library of Congress Catalog Card Number: 84-15638
International Standard Book Number: 0-8361-3373-0
Printed in the United States of America
Design by Alice B. Shetler

90 89 88 87 86 85 84 10 9 8 7 6 5 4 3 2 1

To Mary,
who more than any treatment
or drug,
brought healing.

Contents

Foreword

One of the most difficult problems facing someone with chronic and debilitating illness is that of isolation. Not only physical isolation, but also emotional isolation from friends and family which ultimately leads to isolation from oneself.

With cancer, perhaps more than any other disease, isolation has societal as well as personal ramifications. There is still concern, even in a well educated and sophisticated lay population, that the illness is contagious, and that those with it must be shunned. Physical isolation is also imposed by hospitalization, or by the need to retire from one's profession, often to be bed-bound. The diagnosis of cancer so often conveys with it the feeling that family and friends are powerless to do anything substantive to alter the course of the illness. They are frustrated by feelings of helplessness and hopelessness, which in turn leads to desertion of the patient not only physically but emotionally.

Emotional isolation from family and friends occurs in part from a desire to avoid the fearfully unknown by detachment, and in part because of changing roles within individual relationships. The care-giver is now the care recipient. The once strong father who changed his son's diapers and wiped away his tears now requires assistance from that son to go from bed to bathroom and back, and cries with him as he mourns his own physical disabilities. These role reversals are difficult for both to accept. Since most of us tend to establish our own identity and self-worth in terms of what we can do for and with those we love and respect, such changes are devastating to the patient's sense of self.

Dr. Weaver's book is a statement of the value of continued support from family and friends to anyone with cancer. Such support allows the preservation of self-identity and personal dignity that makes life worth living.

G. S. Edwards, MD
Santa Barbara, California

Author's Preface

I want to share with you a little of my life. Serious illness had always seemed to me to be something that happened to other people. It took some reorientation to face the fact that I had become ill. Many friends helped me to face the situation. They also provided the support that was crucial in my recovery.

I share this story and my viewpoint about it with the hope that it might help others who face cancer. It is not to suggest that my attitudes or actions were in any sense models to be followed. I have rather simply told what they were.

One friend who visited us several times during my illness always remembered to ask my wife, "How is it going with you?" That meant a lot to us, because other family members go through considerable emotional strain when someone is ill. The sick person receives all the attention, but the others take on significantly greater burdens. For that reason each member of my family has written something about his or her reactions to my having cancer. We hope that will be helpful to other family members when illness strikes.

11

When ill, I found that reading about others' experiences was helpful. However, I also found that I lacked the energy needed to do much reading. For that reason, this booklet is deliberately short.

I want to thank my mother who made the line drawings at age 91. They help to express my feelings and situation.

Thanks to the friends who took time to read and make suggestions on the manuscript.

Henry D. Weaver
Santa Barbara, California
December 1983

Confronting the
Big C

1

The Diagnosis

I was aroused by the sound of footsteps in the three-bed ward. As I looked up, Dr. Edwards strode into view. She wore her white coat and was carrying my charts.

"Well, did the biopsy get enough to show anything?" I asked.

"We need to have a long talk," she answered softly as she pulled the curtain around my bed. I knew her words meant something was seriously wrong. I felt shocked. Her words jolted me. Lots of questions raced through my mind. Was I one of those destined to die at an early age? What was ahead? Pain? Difficult treatment? No more walks on the beach?

I had entered the hospital six days before for tests. It was late March and since Valentine's Day I had been following the doctor's orders for complete rest at home.

The problem had started simply enough. I first noticed something amiss the preceding October, when I began losing regularly in tennis to a player with whom I was evenly matched. I knew something was wrong, but I didn't guess how serious the problem would become. I had rarely experienced illness in all my fifty-one years. I had regular exercise, saw a doctor annually for a checkup and in general felt well. However, my feet seemed to be hurting most of the time so I visited a doctor. He felt it was not serious and suggested that probably some cushions in my shoes would solve the problem.

During the next few weeks the small problem seemed to be getting worse. My feet had begun to "flop" when I walked. During Christmas vacation my colleague from the Education Abroad Program of the University of California, Bill Allaway, invited me to play a round of golf at the beautiful La Cumbre Country Club in Santa Barbara. By the end of the first nine I could hardly walk. I was only able to finish the game by sharing an electric cart with another member of the foursome. I would rather not even discuss the score—but then, of course, my game for years has been so bad that I usually don't discuss the score.

Soon afterward I went back to the doctor and he did a more thorough examination. When he hit my knee with his little rubber hammer nothing happened. There was no reflex response. He immediately arranged for a neurologist to see me and I chose Dr. Joseph Blum as the generalist in a group practice to follow my case.

By early January a progressive paralysis was evident and my condition deteriorated quickly so that I soon needed crutches. In less than a month I could only get around in a wheelchair. Those were traumatic steps. I remember distinctly the emotional strain the first time I went to the office with crutches. I sat down with the staff in the Education Abroad Program office and shared with them frankly what the doctors believed the problem was.

The neurologist had diagnosed my difficulty as likely a

disease called the Guillan-Barre syndrome. This condition sometimes resulted from Swine Flu vaccinations. Many physicians believe that it is also caused in some cases by the body's immunological system fighting a virus. Apparently one's own antibodies attack the sheath around nerve fibers causing them to deteriorate. The nerves that give the impulses to the muscles no longer work and paralysis follows. The redeeming feature of the Guillan-Barre syndrome is that the deterioration reverses itself and the paralysis goes away, usually within a month or so.

Dr. Blum followed my case on a daily basis. Several times a week he had me take pulmonary function tests to be sure that the paralysis was not affecting my lungs. After a month he decided that it would be best for me to quit working and have complete rest at home. Each morning I would lie in bed and alternate between naps and the *Los Angeles Times*. We were waiting for the paralysis to reverse itself.

After five weeks of waiting there were no signs that the paralysis was improving. I was discouraged. I looked for some little sign of improvement. Nothing came. As the days had gone by I started to measure how far I could move my feet. It decreased weekly until no movement was possible at all. I watched the strong calves of my legs lose muscle tone and become flabby. I had lost my independence. My wife, Mary, had to do many things for me that I usually did without thinking. I even needed help to get in and out of the bathtub. I began to doubt that the problem was going to start improving.

Also after a few weeks in bed a severe pain began to develop in my back. It bothered me to the extent that I could no longer sit up in bed to read. A friend loaned me some prism glasses so that I could lie flat and read, but if you have ever tried to read a large newspaper that way, you know it is less than satisfactory.

As I lay in bed day after day nothing improved. I began to doubt that my condition would ever change. Mary would bring my breakfast before going off to work and then I would nap and read, nap and read, and nap and read some more until she came home for lunch. After her half-hour lunch break it was nap and read, nap and read, nap and read some more as I watched the sunlight fade and waited for her to come through the door again after work. Nothing improved and my muscles became weaker.

After some inquiries we learned that one of the world experts on the Guillan-Barre syndrome was at the University of California in San Francisco. Dr. Blum called and made an appointment for me to see him. Bill Allaway arranged to go with me on the plane. However, the day before the trip, Dr. Blum decided to take one last round of x-rays and see if he could find anything. He saw a small abnormality in a vertebra.

He decided to follow that up with extensive tests and so had me admitted to the hospital instead of my going to San Francisco. An impressive succession of specialists examined me. Each specialist took time to describe the tests they proposed and the possible meaning of the results. The first inkling I had that cancer could be involved was when Dr. Georgia Edwards appeared one evening and said she was an oncologist. I probably showed a little amazement since I thought she said "gynecologist."

In any case, she quickly explained that she was a tumor specialist. One of the tests they did was a myelogram. In that test some spinal fluid is removed and replaced by a dye. The patient is then tilted at various angles on a table while the doctor watches with a fluoroscope. In my case when the dye reached a vertebra fairly high on my back (called the T-6 vertebra), it was blocked and could go no further. The x-rays of the vertebra showed it resembling a piece of Swiss cheese.

The doctors discussed with me the possibility of taking a biopsy. That would tell whether or not there was a malignancy or an infection involved but it also had the possibility of causing paralysis if the biopsy needle struck the spinal cord. We decided, therefore, to use an alternate approach called a "thin-needle biopsy" which would not injure the cord if the needle hit it, but also carried a possibility that not enough material could be collected to make a diagnosis.

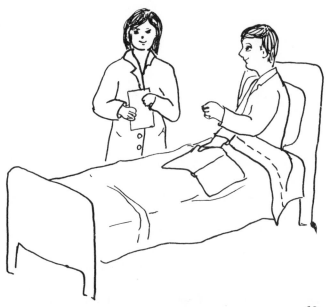

As Dr. Edwards stood by my bed she explained that an adequate sample had been collected and that the cause of the problem in the vertebra was cancer. Cancer! The word conveyed a myriad of images. My father had cancer of the colon at age 75 and it was successfully removed surgically. But I had also lost several friends to the disease. I knew if cancer could be detected in time, often it could be controlled or cured. I also knew it could kill me. I asked what kind of cancer mine was, and what could be done about it. Did I face surgery? Could the cancer be isolated and removed? Dr. Edwards explained that my kind of cancer could be treated by radiation with almost one hundred percent assurance that it would be completely irradicated from the vertebra. Good news—there would not need to be a painful back operation!

What kind of malignancy was it? She explained that it was an adenocarcinoma, a kind that could not have arisen in the vertebra. That meant there was a primary cancer in some other organ and cancerous cells were obviously circulating through my bloodstream. Nothing seemed worse to me. Obviously, even if we found the primary source and cut it out, cancer had already spread throughout my system. In my mind was the question, "How long will I have?"

Knowing that the myelogram showed pressure on the spinal cord, she leveled with me: "You probably will never be able to walk again." All that registered in my mind was, "You will never walk again."

"That's pretty heavy," I murmured as I sunk deeper into the mattress. I thought about my fifty-one years of life so far. I felt at peace if my time had come. I couldn't say I had been cheated in life if this was the end. I had a family I was proud of and I felt good about my interaction with them over the years. I had seen more corners of the earth and enjoyed more variety of experiences than many people in their eighties. But I really enjoyed life and activities too much to want it to end.

But now it seemed it would end. Why? Why? I'm a guy who likes to ski, play tennis, and walk. But I won't ever walk again! It was bad enough developing a limp when I walked around campus. During the last month it was embarrassing to meet strangers from my wheelchair. But I knew the symptoms would reverse and sometime later I would see those same people and I would be walking, fast and surefooted as I always had. But now she was saying I had cancer. I might die. If not that, she was saying I would never walk again.

"I will walk by the first of May," I informed her, and to this day I am not sure why I said that.

2

Attitude and Expectation

Recently I entered the University of California tennis courts at noon with a friend. I still had braces on both feet and could not move about quickly enough to give my friend a first-class game—or to take a set from him. When I entered the court, the fellow to whom I had been losing regularly as I became ill came over to welcome me back on the courts and to wish me well. He surprised me by what he said. Like many of us, he had a deep-seated fear of cancer. Knowing that I had been side-lined with the disease but now stood there with a racket in my hand gave him a new confidence. He said that he is no longer afraid; he knows it is possible to conquer "the big C."

An increasing number of studies show that he is right and that our attitudes and expectations have a lot to do with recovery.

Two days after the diagnosis, my wife, Mary, came in as usual during her lunch break from the laboratory where she works as a technologist. She gave me a mimeographed research report. At the top of the first page, Dr. Wilcox, who worked in her lab, had written:

"You might want to give this to Hank when you think he is ready." That report became one of a whole series of links in a chain that saved my life.

The report was written by an oncologist-psychologist husband-and-wife team, the Simontons. The part of the paper that struck me most forcibly was a research report in which they had studied 152 patients at the Fort Worth Veterans' Hospital where they worked. Each of these patients had cancer which gave a life expectancy of six months. The staff at the hospital ranked the patients in terms of their attitude on a 5-point scale from double minus to double plus. Eighteen months later they evaluated the condition of the patients. Remarkably all of those that had plus or double plus attitudes were at work. All of those with double minus attitudes were dead. For a chemist like myself, used to drawing conclusions from empirical research, the effect of that paper was powerful.

Dr. Edwards suggested I obtain their book, *Getting Well Again*. I read it. They mention another book in their paper, *The Will to Live* by Arnold Hutchnecker. Mary went out and purchased the book for me. It's well worth reading. He cites case after case in which the expectation by the patient of getting well appeared to be the crucial difference. He arrives at the straightforward conclusion that "you die when you want to die." Barring some, but not all, accidents, "you do not die until you are willing to." Whether or not his conclusion is valid, case histories and evidence he cites are overwhelming. It became clear that one of the factors which would enable me to get well again was my own attitude, my expectation of recovery, my own will to live.

I became convinced that I was going to live. I decided that I would walk again. My friends and family acted as if

23

they expected me to regain health.

It is clear that there is more involved in the effect of attitude than some flimsy notion or wish. Our emotions have concrete, measurable physiological effects on our physical bodies. We know this at some simple levels. Tears, real salty physical tears, come out of our tear ducts when we are sad. That is a physical response to our emotions. Our "mouths water" when mentally we anticipate a delicious meal. Thirty years ago at our wedding I measured my pulse just before walking into the ceremony. It was 120. There was no physical activity to account for that, just my emotional state. The secretion of glands that occurs during sexual activity are partially due to physical stimulation, but also strongly related to mental and emotional expectations.

Hans Selye, a Canadian biochemist, has written extensively about stress, including emotional stress, and its effects on the body. He has measured the flow of secretions from the endocrine glands caused by emotional reactions.

It is entirely reasonable, therefore, to expect that our emotional side, our attitudes and our expectations, will have physiological consequences in fighting disease, including cancer. We don't know the exact mechanism or all of the details of the process, but neither do I know the mechanism that makes me shed tears when I am sad.

The Simontons have developed a procedure that they believe enables the mind to assist the body in dealing with cancer or other diseases. I attempted to use the process that they describe in their book, *Getting Well Again*. It involves the formation of an image. The first step is to relax and imagine yourself in pleasant surroundings. I imagined myself at the Goleta Beach. I could hear the gentle sound of the waves and see the gulls flying overhead. The sun was shining and the sky clear. The waves were crashing with a big spray on the point. Boats floated at anchor nearby.

One is then supposed to imagine something to represent the white blood cells attacking the cancer cells in the bloodstream and destroying them. I imagined the white cells as little soldiers armed and ready to shoot the evil cancer cells when they appeared. I even equipped the good guys with white hats and the bad guys with black hats. Unfortunately, it didn't work. I am a pacifist, and even to save my life I couldn't have the nice fellows shooting the bad ones with the black hats. I changed the image and saw the white cells as porpoises with little white sailor caps devouring the bad fish. They gobbled them up and I mentally cheered them on.

The chemotherapy I was receiving consisted of three different drugs. These I saw as animated red, white, and blue circles that ensnared the bad cells and shoved them into the gutter.

Incidentally, if you find it hard to believe that your emotions affect your body, let me suggest chemotherapy. I received the medicine by injection once a week for two weeks and then went for two weeks without it while the white count in my blood regenerated. There were some definite physiological side effects. My hair came out, sense of my taste changed, and I experienced nausea for a few days after each treatment.

However, I also developed some psychological conditioned responses that put me in the class with Pavlov's famous dog. Both Dr. Edwards and her nurse, Donna, are attractive women, intelligent, and pleasant to chat with. If you think psychological conditioning has no physiological consequences, how do you explain the embarrassing fact that when I would go into their office, *before* they gave the actual injection, the sight of these beautiful women would cause me to throw up? Fortunately, after the chemotherapy was discontinued, so did my abnormal behavior.

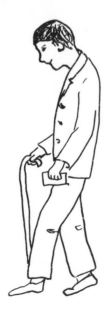

I am convinced that my declaration that I would walk again was a significant factor in regaining the use of my legs. The destruction of the cancer cells in my back was accompanied by the slow physiological recovery of nerves and muscles. However, there was a constant need to consciously do something about it. Once I had declared my intent to walk again, the goal became an obsession with me. I thought about it frequently. I fantasized about it. I watched how others walked. I considered how I used to ski and ride on a unicycle. Those were acts of balance. Why shouldn't I be able to walk—which is also an act of balance—even if my paralyzed feet were held rigid by plastic braces?

My commitment to walk again gave me some of the courage to leave the wheelchair and strike out on crutches. I remember distinctly the day I left the wheelchair at home for the first time and used the crutches to go to the office from the car where Mary dropped me off. It also took some courage when the physical therapist told me it would be okay to drive the car again. I won't forget the day I left the crutches in the car and used only a cane. I remember the day I left the cane at home and walked with no support. I was a bit wobbly, but it was progress.

The expectation of recovery was a vital part of the process.

3

Sally

Christmas, 1979, was my first visit to Santa Barbara. Mom and Dad had moved there that fall. Don and I were the only kids home that Christmas. Judy was in Spain on a junior year abroad program and Deb had flown over to spend the holiday with her. I was working in a bank in Goshen, Indiana, at that time and a two-week vacation in California was great. Dad gave us the "25-cent tour" of all the sights. I roamed the beach looking for shells; we drove up into the mountains to go skiing. Mom and Dad seemed to be enjoying the new location, the weather, their jobs, new friends.

There was a minor, scarcely heard, dissonant note to the holiday. Dad's feet were bothering him. They were numb and prevented him from doing much walking, or from controlling his skis properly. He had been to the doctor, who thought it might be that a new pair of shoes were too tight. Dad had stopped wearing them but the numbness stayed. Don and I returned to Goshen, mildly curious as to what could be wrong.

During the next months the calls kept coming: Dad's feet were getting worse; his fingers grew numb; he couldn't type; he couldn't write. The muscles in his feet seemed to be deteriorating; he couldn't walk without crutches; he couldn't walk *with* crutches. "They" thought it might be due to the Guillan-Barre syndrome.

People in Goshen had begun to hear that all was not well with Dad. Friends of his from Goshen College, from the business community, and from the College Church would stop Don and Deb on campus, or come to my bank window and ask, "Anything new on your father?"

Most of us had never heard of the Guillan-Barre syndrome. "Well, it's a progressive deterioration of the peripheral nervous system," we tried to explain. "It should continue getting worse for a while and then turn around and go back to normal."

But it didn't. It was a frustrating time. The illness was at a standstill and there was nothing to be done. News that they had found cancer came almost as a relief. At last—something concrete. Finally there was something to be treated, steps that could be taken to fight the problem—spot radiation for the vertebra, physical therapy for his feet, chemotherapy, and the like. Nothing is worse than the helplessness of feeling that nothing really can be done.

It probably helped that I didn't have much cancer "baggage." Of course, it is more or less in the societal air—everyone knows what cancer is. If nothing else, they know that rats stuffed with bacon, or soda pop, or whatever, tend to get it. But no one close to me had ever died from cancer. The word itself was not a black-clad messenger bearing inevitable death. It was definitely a cause for concern, but I don't remember agonizing over "Why does Dad have to die?" I didn't think he would, though I do remember wondering if my (hypothetical)

29

husband and children would have a chance to know my father.

Several factors added to the non-worried attitude. One was distance. With half a continent between us it was hard to grasp that Dad was seriously ill. It didn't seem real. I wasn't there, watching him become bedfast, undergoing series of tests, growing gaunt. Over the phone he sounded much like he always had, filling us in on details, or subjecting us to his latest joke.

Dad's attitude was another factor. We knew he and Mom would let us know what they knew, when they knew it. And Dad's positive approach was contagious. Shortly before I came out to Santa Barbara at the beginning of May, I tried to explain to a medical student friend the imaging Dad was using, and his attitude in general. I got the impression that she thought he was simply not facing up to the reality of the situation. I don't believe that Dad's approach was a denial of facts. Dad knew what the facts were. His inquisitive nature led him to probe into things and ask his doctors many questions. He knew what the situation was but chose to face it positively.

This is in line with his whole approach to life—reaching out to it, enjoying it, always having an alternative plan ready if the first one doesn't pan out. I don't mean to imply that he was always cheerful, never complaining. While I was in Goshen, communicating mostly with phone calls, he generally projected a strong positive attitude, as did Mom. When I was in California, even though by then he was already on the road to recovery, I noticed the day-to-day smaller complaints. He tired quickly and had to go to bed early. Food didn't taste right and the daily pills he needed to take during his two-week "period" caused a constant grumble. The nausea brought about by chemotherapy and his psychosomatic reactions to it were hard for him to take. On the whole, though, it was a sort of surface complaining, like yelling "ouch" when you stub your toe. His basic approach to his illness was not one of complaining or despair, but "I can lick this."

I believe there was yet a third factor affecting the attitudes of the whole family, though it is a difficult one to assess. Many people were praying for Dad—and they were also praying for the rest of us. Perhaps they took our burden of worry and fear upon themselves so that we were freed for other things. For a variety of reasons unconnected with Dad's illness, that period was a particularly low point for me. I was struggling with a number of problems and uncertainties—my job didn't seem worthwhile; I couldn't decide what direction to head with training or career; I felt surrounded by happy couples; a church committee I was chairing was at a stalemate. Many little things added up. It is important to face the possibility of death and work through the ramifications, but because of the other factors weighing on me at the time, it might have been more than I could handle.

A series of episodes epitomize for me the determination and rapidity of Dad's return to health. During the month of May all four of us children returned to Santa Barbara. Because of our schedules, we all came back at different times, arriving at weekly intervals. The airport is only a fifteen-minute drive from home, so it was easy for both Mom and Dad to come pick us up.

I was the first one home. I flew from Chicago to San Francisco and hopped a puddle-jumper to Santa Barbara. As I walked from the plane to the Spanish white walls and red tiles of the terminal, I could see Mom waiting at the

31

gate. Dad had stayed in the car; his wheelchair was in the trunk.

Deb came a week later, back from a marine biology class in Florida. Dad was getting used to his half-crutches by then, and with their help he came to the arrival gate. Deb could see him waiting as soon as she got off the plane.

Don came the following week. Again, Dad pushed himself. Leaving his crutches at home, he made his way into the airport waiting area with a cane.

Judy was the last to arrive, returning from her year in Spain. Except for Deb, who had been with her at Christmas, none of us had seen her for a year. While the rest of us had been able to talk with Mom and Dad frequently by phone, Judy had heard about Dad's illness mostly by letter and tape. Dad wanted to reassure her immediately that things were improving. He walked out to meet her, using only a hand on Mom's shoulder for support.

By the time I left for Goshen, six weeks after I came, he

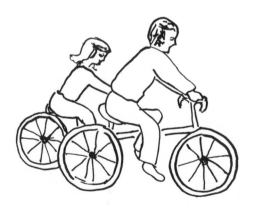

was riding his bike to work. A friend had loaned him a bicycle-exerciser earlier, and he had slowly been building up his strength. Then he tried the bike, with two of us on each side for security. Finally, one day I accompanied him on the bike ride from home to the university. For the most part it is a pleasant easy ride that takes you past the Goleta slough and beach. The last lap, the hill from the beach to the campus, was the challenge. Dad had figured he might have to get off the bike and walk. But he kept chugging away, and got to the top a lot less out of breath than I was.

Because of the rapidity of Dad's return to activity and because of the ongoing all-clear records from the CAT scans, I'm always a little taken by surprise when people ask with great concern how Dad is doing. It is under-standable—not everyone who knew him in Goshen has kept up on all the details. Two years after he went back to work full time and a year and a half after he was walking nearly normally and had gone off chemotherapy, I had someone ask me recently how he was doing and if he was out of a wheelchair yet.

Well, yes. The concern and sympathy I feel in the question almost seems misplaced. Dad? Oh, yeah, he had cancer once.

4

The Cancer Model

What was taking place in my body? What happens physically in any cancer? To understand the answer to those questions, it's important to understand the nature of any scientific answer. Science does not lead to answers with one hundred percent assurance that they are correct. What we do in science is to build models. The goal is simply that the model be useful. It does not need to be unique.

In my own case there was disagreement between various physicians involved on exactly what was happening. In the more general sense, a variety of models are being proposed and tested by scientists engaged in research, to explain how cancer develops and how it might be cured. In that context the explanation I want to give should be seen as one way to pull together the various facets in this case, but it is certainly not the only possible explanation or working model to explain them.

In my case apparently a form of cancer developed in some gland or soft tissue of my body. This was called the primary source and its location was not detected. Cells from the primary source entered the bloodstream and some of these lodged and began their uncontrolled reproduction in a vertebra high in my backbone, identified as the "T-6 vertebra." This was the secondary location of cancer.

Cancer in a bone such as this eats away the calcium deposit and leaves the vertebra mottled with holes. In my case the x-rays and CAT scans clearly showed this vertebra to have lots of holes and the tissue around it to be swollen. That easily explained the pain I had in my back and the fact that when dye was injected into my spinal column it was blocked and could not flow past the T-6 vertebra. But how can one explain from that the numbness and paralysis that came to my hands, legs, and feet?

Apparently there is not a universally accepted explanation for that phenomenon although it is occasionally observed in cancer. One possible explanation is that the same thing happened in this case that occurs in the Guillan-Barre syndrome, the original diagnosis. According to the *Handbook of Neurology,* there are two theories for the cause of this disease. One sees it as a side effect of a virus infection and the other as the result of an immunization shot. Some people became ill with the Guillan-Barre syndrome following vaccination for Swine Flu. In these cases it is assumed that the antibodies produced from this stimulus attack the nerve fibers, damaging or destroying them. It is generally believed that in cancer the body's immunological system is activated and so it would seem reasonable that if my body was fighting the cancer, it may have generated antibodies that attacked my nerves.

The fact that these nerves have since regenerated is consistent with that model, since peripheral nerve tissue

35

(the nerves out in the arms and legs) do regenerate while central nervous system tissue (such as that in the spinal cord) does not regenerate, at least not after much time has lapsed. That is why the doctor thought I probably would never walk again. There was evidence that the malignancy was putting pressure on my spinal column and possibly damaging it.

While the different physicians involved are not in complete agreement on whether or not there was damage to the spinal cord, I am convinced that there was not. Observations such as the loss of reflexes in my knees and the symmetrical nature of the paralysis and loss of sensation are consistent with that point of view.

What about the fact that extensive testing has not revealed the primary source of my cancer? Assuming that the diagnosis was correct and that a primary source existed, then either the physicians have not looked at the right place with a sensitive enough probe to detect it or it has gone away. They have looked, with the best tools available. There were x-rays and sputum tests for the lungs, biopsies of the prostate, examination of the upper and lower G.I. tract, and complete body CAT scans. They tried every test I had ever heard about, with the exception of a PAP smear!

One possible explanation is that my own immunological system took care of the malignancy. Another possibility is that the chemotherapy I received stopped it. Something I read one day while waiting for the doctor in her office suggests a possibility. In one study an examination was made of the prostate of all males who died for *any cause* in a given hospital. In 14 percent of the cases the person was found to have cancer of the prostate. In only a few of those malignancies could a trained pathologist detect the cancer by examining the prostate without the microscopic slide.

I am told that in another study, examinations were made of the tissue taken from the breasts of all women who died from *any cause*. About 20 percent of them were found to have cancer of the breast. Allowing for the fact that cancer would only be detected when the slide was taken from the right location within the organ, it seems reasonable to assume that a fourth or a fifth of healthy people have microscopic cancer that is being held in control by their bodies.

I find that a reasonable model. I assume that I have had a microscopic cancer in some organ for many years. I assume that either due to my own immunological system or to the effect of the chemotherapy it is again dormant. I don't expect to hear from it again, but it's not impossible that I might. I'll keep having regular checkups, thank you.

Obviously, if many of us are walking around with dormant cancer, an important part of the model is to understand what might cause it to get out of control. A growing number of scientists believe that in many cases stress and psychological factors are involved. Many cases have been observed in which after the death of a person, his or her spouse developed cancer within six months to a year. Other writers note that cancer is not unusual following forced retirement or some other highly stressful situation. I do not know of enough studies with adequate control groups to make that a commonly accepted phenomenon, but I find it a reasonable part of the model.

In my own case, cancer followed a number of stressful changes. I had left a job that I thoroughly enjoyed, and felt fully accepted in; I had sold a house that we liked and

37

which had a lot of my own labor in it. We had moved to California, a long way from our Indiana home. Our four children had gone off to college or new jobs and for the first time Mary and I found ourselves alone in a too-quiet, too-tidy house. Although I liked my new job and the people I worked with, the city and the state to which I had moved were new to me. Those changes—by any-body's accounting—represented a lot of stress.

Whether or not those factors were important in this particular case, the model suggests that whatever other cause might be involved in cancer, good mental health, the enjoyment of life, and the reduction of stress are im-portant in controlling or preventing it.

Research seems to indicate that a variety of things en-courage cancer. Smoking or inhaling asbestos increases the probability of lung cancer. Too much sun is impli-cated in some skin cancers and a variety of foods and chemicals have been assigned responsibility for other cancers. How do these things fit into the model? What emerges is similar to our understanding of disease caused by bacteria. Certain bacteria have been identified as responsible for certain diseases. Yet we know that when a group of people are exposed to a particular strain of disease-causing bacteria, some of them get ill and some do not. Obviously there is more involved than a given in-fection resulting from exposure to a particular type of bac-teria. One of those additional factors is the working of the body's immunological system to fight foreign agents such as bacteria. Many think stress is another factor that helps determine whether or not the body becomes ill when exposed to bacteria.

In a parallel way the model of cancer that emerges is this. Causative agents, many of which are not adequately identified, are received in the body and are capable of initiating cancer. The body's immunological system fights these stimuli. Stress, attitudes, and one's general mental condition are factors, but not the only factors, in how successful the body will be in fighting these stimuli. When the body is not able to control the malignancy, surgical removal, chemotherapy, radiation, mental imagery, and other techniques may assist the body in fighting the malignancy. In a growing number of cases, the body, with the help of these other tools, is winning the battle.

Our society needs to change its picture of cancer. The press talks about the "cancer victim" as someone who has contracted a "dread disease." We aren't treated with medicine but rather with "chemotherapy." We seem not to be aware of the tremendous strides that have been made in the last few years in the treatment of cancer. Our minds have grown used to definitive, spectacular breakthroughs such as we saw when the Salk vaccine essentially eliminated polio. We need also to realize that much progress has been made with cancer, little by little.

Recently I saw a news release claiming that until four years before the time I was diagnosed as having cancer, practically all the people with cancer of the backbone died from the illness. The release claimed that with the use of radiation, most if not all of the same cases are now adequately being restored. Whether or not my own cancer in a vertebra was the same as that discussed in the news article I don't know, but I do know that radiation came to my rescue and that on seeing the release I had a profound sense of gratitude for being alive.

It might help us to think of cancer today as we do a disease such as diabetes. There are many similarities between cancer and diabetes. Both decrease life expectancy, both can give complications to other ailments, neither is contagious, both can frequently be controlled by medicine. However, our society has come to terms with diabetes in a mature way that we have not yet applied to cancer.

Let's *expect* the person who contracts cancer to be able to deal with it and continue to lead a productive life. In more cases than not, our expectation will be realized!

5

Support Group

In late March 1980 when Dr. Edwards told me that I would perhaps never walk again, I replied that I would walk by the first of May. No one was more surprised by that utterance than myself. It was completely out of character. I have a high regard for physicians. Over the years hundreds of students from my chemistry classes have gome on to become medical doctors. I am fully aware that they differ widely in their abilities. Many times I have faced the question on the recommendation sheet to a medical school that asks whether or not I would want this person to be my own physician if he or she should finish medical school. There have been some cases when the answer was "no." However, even with those misgivings, I find that the doctors who treat me are either well respected or I soon change physicians.

The internist in charge of my case was Dr. Blum. He is very bright, compassionate, and also secure enough to say so when he doesn't know something. He had selected my oncologist, Dr. Edwards. She examined me in the hospital at about the same time that a dozen other doctors examined me, and I noticed that she picked up details and related bits of information that no one else caught. More than that, she treated me as an intellectual equal. She discussed with me the tests that were being made and the possible outcomes. The dynamics of the situation were clear. When she indicated that I had probable damage of the spinal cord and would likely never walk again, I should have believed her. Instead I talked back. I made a simple declaratory statement that I would walk again.

On reflection, I am convinced making that statement had a lot to do with the fact that on the 30th of April I began walking with the aid of crutches. I had a strong drive to get back to work. There were only a few times that I thought I would not recover. I am convinced that this positive expectation, this positive attitude, was absolutely crucial in regaining my strength and returning to work. Where did that strength come from? What made me positive?

No simple answer is sufficient, but I am convinced that a major factor was the support that I received from others. In a short span of time I realized how incredibly rich I was at the point that counted most—friends. Less than six months earlier, I had left my job as provost and professor of chemistry at Goshen College in Indiana. I had been on the staff for twenty-two years and felt I was doing a good job. The faculty of about a hundred and twenty-five people were close friends of mine. The community in which I lived was small and there were lots of interactions with other people. The Mennonite church I attended gave high priority to interacting and caring with other people. The local Rotary Club had a hundred-plus members whom I knew on a first name basis and saw at least once a week.

But when I became ill, I was in Santa Barbara, California. I'd had less than six months to make new acquaintances and friendships. But suddenly there was a virtual explosion of friendship and caring. I remember especially one three-week period when my spirits were at a low point. What we thought was Guillan-Barre syndrome was not responding as it should. My condition was getting worse week by week and we didn't know what it was.

During that three-week period there was only one night in which I did not receive a call from one of my colleagues at Goshen College. Some evenings as many as four or five would call me. Mary comes from a family with ten children and in my own there were five. These siblings are scattered widely throughout the United States and every one of them called at one time or another to give me support.

A former student, Carl Keener, now a psychiatrist in Denver, sent me Norman Cousins' book, *The Anatomy of an Illness.* A brother-in-law and his wife, Aaron and Bertie Eby, who knew my convoluted sense of humor sent me several books of limericks.

As one would anticipate, I received a lot of strength and encouragement from my immediate family. All four of our children were away from home at the time. Don and Deb were students at Goshen College; Judy was in a junior year abroad program in Seville, Spain; and Sally was working in a bank in Goshen, Indiana. Their calls and letters expressed a depth of relationship that one tends not to talk about in more normal times.

Mary took on the burden of help and support with an attitude of love and care that had no sense of martyrdom to it. I remember distinctly one dark day when I was con-

43

vinced that I would probably never recover. I was not bitter about death, but clearly disappointed.

From my bed I could see my closet and the thought struck me that I would never need to buy any additional clothes. It was a morbid thought. Any additional suits or shirts that I might get would simply be a problem to dispose of after I was gone. I told Mary about that thought. Later as my attitude shifted to a more positive one, I resolved that even though we were short of cash, one of my early acts upon getting out of bed would be to purchase a navy blue blazer and khaki pants which I had been wanting. When my birthday came in early May, both of us had tears in our eyes when she gave me a blue blazer and khaki pants. It was more than a gift of clothing; it was a statement by both the giver and the recipient of faith in life.

Because of my work we had lived in several other parts of the world for periods of a year or less. In administration of the Goshen College overseas programs I had made many friends in other countries. As word of my illness spread I received cards and letters from Nepal, Poland, Peru, Costa Rica, and other places. Protestant, Catholic, Jewish, and Hindu friends wrote to say they were praying for me. When because of my illness I missed a board meeting of the Council on International Educational Exchange in New York, I received a card signed by each of the people there. That had deep meaning for me.

I also discovered a lot of support from new friends. The Education Abroad Program Senate Committee of the University of California sent me a letter of wishes and prayers when they met. Only about two weeks before I became ill we had begun to attend the Goleta Presbyterian Church. The pastor began to call on me regularly and was most supportive. Another member of the church, Tom Allin, who had also received radiation therapy for a back problem, came to see me and share his experience. Charlotte McDonald, who has an unusual gift for growing flowers, sent me some regularly in the hospital and to my home after my release. As I began attending church again, first in a wheelchair, then on crutches, then with a cane, and finally with only the help of my braces, a dozen different people whose names I had not yet learned took time to cheer me on and encourage me.

The staff with whom I had worked only a few months were incredible. As my ability to walk decreased with the onset of the problem and I went to a cane, crutches, and finally a wheelchair, the staff took it in stride. They showed support without condescension. When I returned to work the same support was there as I moved from a wheelchair to crutches, a cane, and finally without mechanical aid. As I began to be able to walk, but was still not able to run, Roger Horton, the vice chancellor for

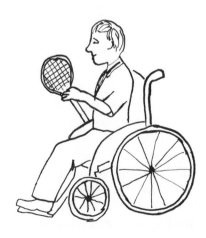

financial affairs, offered to begin hitting tennis balls to me and arranged both handicap singles and doubles play, even though the quality of my play was dubious. That led to some interesting situations. Even though I could walk reasonably well and could stand for a period which enabled me to play tennis, I still found the handicap parking space near my office a major asset preventing the need to walk too far. When you get out of a car parked in a handicap zone with a tennis racket in hand, you are the object of a few stares and as a matter of fact, feel a little guilty!

When I was hospitalized and immediately afterward, help came from many sources locally. Our friends Gerry and Abe Freisen came over once a week and mowed our lawn. Delores Kelly, who was in charge of the laboratory in which Mary worked, let her adjust her schedule so she could visit me every day at noon as well as in the evening. Bill Allaway, my immediate supervisor, came to see me daily. Numerous members of the staff visited me in the hospital. After I was released from the hospital, my secretary, Judy Messick, coordinated arrangements so that one of the staff was available to pick me up at home and take me in for radiation treatment each day.

A number of friends went to considerable lengths to give me support. Lawrence Burkholder, the president of Goshen College with whom I had worked closely during the preceding ten years, deviated from his route on a trip to stop and see me. Richard Strasser, a neighbor with whom I had shared trips in the past, came to see me and indicated that he would fly out any time that it would make a significant difference. My brother called to see if he should cancel a trip to Florida to visit me instead. A friend, John Bender, who is a specialist in physical medicine now living in Utah, offered to stop and see me. A number of other people, including Willard Krabill, who had been my personal physician in Goshen for many years, went out of their way on other trips to call on me in Santa Barbara. Chet and Gerry Raber, friends from college days, came to visit. Gerry, who had faced many of my problems as a result of polio, helped me understand a lot about living with a physical handicap. Chet, a psychologist, spent hours on the phone helping me sort things out.

What did all of that have to do with getting well? It gave me a clear message, "We care about you." People cared whether I lived or died. People cared whether or not I could walk and do the things I wanted to do. Whether or not they were using the words, people were saying they loved me. That made me want to live. That made me want to walk. That increased my drive to want to play tennis and ski and swim and do all the things I enjoyed. I am convinced that this support was as important as the radiation and the chemotherapy in pulling me back to health.

Another important support group was my physicians. None of them ever used the term "holistic medicine" to describe what was going on, but every one of them practiced it. The doctors worked *with* me not *on* me. Each of them interacted with me as a person, not just an object of his or her practice. Dr. Blum frequently took time to explain what was going on. He made sure I saw the x-rays and showed me the points my untrained eye did not catch. Each specialist took time to describe proposed tests to Mary and me and to tell us the meaning of different possible results. Dr. Edwards explained the dangers when she raised the possibility of taking a biopsy of the vertebra. She shared with us the issues involved in deciding whether to continue the chemotherapy after a year. Drs. Edwards and Blum invited me to sit in when my case was a part of the "grand rounds" for discussion by other physicians.

This attitude was important to me. It was important because obviously the choices were often not black and white and my confidence in their decisions increased when I knew what they were considering. It was important because I was a person about whom they cared. I was not just a number being treated. Since they leveled with me in good news or bad, I knew I could depend on them. I never wondered if they were keeping something sinister from me. They were caring humans—not just technicians. They told jokes and they laughed at mine. They had families, avocations, and many interests. They were also technically competent and both that competence and their humanness helped to heal me.

6

Mary

Three years later as I contemplate Hank's illness and my reactions to it, I think of several stages we went through.

The first stage began when Hank's symptoms became definable and body chemistries and physical changes could be measured, resulting in a diagnosis of a classic textbook case of Guillan-Barre syndrome. This did not scare me. It was depressing and saddening to know that someone I loved was being put through the frightening experience of increasing paralysis, but reading about the prognosis of Guillan-Barre, I was confidently optimistic in feeling that Hank's illness would continue to follow the classic pattern—reversing itself and improving until Hank was once again as "good as new," or as close as a 51-year-old can be to "new."

The second stage began when there was no textbook recovery and the days blurred into weeks and weeks began to change to months. This was probably the most frightening time, knowing that things were not going as they should; wondering, during the late hours of the night and the alone times in the car on my way to work, or on errands of family responsibilities, wondering what was really happening. Something was wrong with the recovery system of Hank's body. What was going on or what was not functioning inside that body?

I watched Hank growing weaker and weaker, the slow advancement of the paralysis as it persistently crept from toes to ankles to legs, from fingertips to finger joints and into the hands. He went from cane to crutches to wheelchair. Finally Hank could not get in or out of bed without my help. He could barely hold a pencil to write his name or punch a typewriter key. The sensitivity to touch in his extremities was excruciatingly painful. Possibly the saddest thing to watch happening was the loss of his ability to write or type—this husband of mine who lived with words and formed those words into ideas and plans of action, smashing them out on the typewriter as they developed.

I floundered some at this time. Anger and despair sometimes washed over me. We had just moved to one of

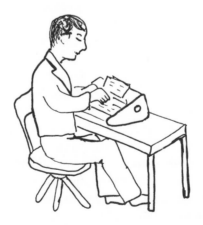

the most beautiful spots on earth and we could not enjoy it together. Angry, because I was forced to take over Hank's role in many ways—to be the initiator, the instigator, the strong organizer. This was not me, but I knew I had to become this just now as we looked for answers. Angry, because even though I had worked for years as a medical technologist, California would not recognize my national accreditation and I was being forced to take, along with all other medical technologists moving into the state, the California state board exams. This meant I had to put any time I could spare into studying for the exam only a few weeks away.

Actually I was not perpetually angry. That usually came only at the times of most frustration. Sometimes frightened, sometimes worried, would probably describe my emotions more often during this period. Fortunately, my apprehension was constantly being eased by the shared concern and support of family far and wide, of old friends in Indiana, of new ones in Santa Barbara, by the flexibility of my supervisor allowing me to adjust my schedule to the needs of my husband. Hope was frequently talked into being.

The third phase involved Hank's hospital stay and treatment following. I have just said I feel the preceding phase was the most frightening time for me. But the day Hank told me during my lunch break with him that the biopsy revealed cancer, I was frightened into numbness. As I drove to the hospital that noon I was apprehensive because I knew Hank would probably have the report. I remember we both cried when he told me. We made conversation, thoughts that moved in on us with no answers yet. What treatment were they discussing? Where was the primary site?

When will we call the children to let them know? We latched on to that. It was our philosophy always to inform the children first and to pass along to them all the information we knew. We had told them they were not to worry about rumors they might hear, because as soon as we knew something we would let them know. When at one point a rumor started making the rounds in Goshen that Hank had a brain tumor, they began to fear that we might have reneged on our stated intent.

So even in our numbness that day we knew we needed to let our children know immediately and then tell key members of our larger family. We could phone them that evening. I drove back to work, unable to think beyond that one fact—Hank had cancer.

I told my supervisor as soon as I arrived at the lab. "Do you want to take the rest of the day off?" she asked. I knew immediately I did not. I did not want to be at home alone with that numbness. I wanted to be doing something, something to occupy my mind on other things, to move me through the day.

During the afternoon our pastor called me. He had been keeping close contact during these days. He had been to see Hank. He knew the diagnosis. He wanted me to know he was available if I needed anything. He would pray.

"Yes," I said, "please do. I am not able to pray today. You will have to do it for us."

That numbing fright did not last beyond that first day. When the problem was known, the medical personnel at the hospital immediately swung into action. Streams of tests were conducted to determine the primary site of the lesion; radiation was begun; a drug program was instituted. Hank was in the thick of it, involving himself and being involved by the doctors to work at whatever needed to be done to get well. I saw and felt the expertise of the medical staff. There was a plan of action that could be carried out. Confidence and great hope came with this. I knew that cancer did not automatically mean death. I knew that many cancer patients get well. There was hope.

The one person who generated that hope and confidence in me more than any other was Hank himself. His determination was infectious. He read books to help him deal with the psychological aspects of having cancer and vigorously applied what he was learning to himself. He set goals and made every attempt to reach them. Usually he did. I was amazed at the rapidity of his recovery, and I still am as I look back on it.

7

The Role of Prayer

Dr. Blum, the internist treating me, remarked about a year after I had been hospitalized, "Your recovery is really miraculous." At the time I was hospitalized, I counted one day more than a dozen different churches that I had been told were praying for my recovery. Numerous friends in various parts of the world sent notes that they were remembering me at mass or in the temple. Many friends, and particularly the members of my family, told me they were praying. Did these prayers have anything to do with my recovery?

My answer is a simple one of faith. Yes. But, you may ask, where do the other things fit in? The excellent medical team? The good medical facilities? The support of friends for a positive mental attitude? I really don't know, but let me share my perspective about it.

When you ask "How does prayer fit into the scheme of things?" or "How do you know prayer works?" you are asking questions that presuppose a scientific model of thought. One perspective of mine is an assumption about the limitations in scientific models. I have already mentioned that in science we build models to explain things and then test the models by experiments, or observations. If we are thinking critically about what we are doing as scientists, we do not assume that our models are complete. We assume that we are involving a limited number of variables in the model. We recognize that other factors may be involved. We limit our observations to the things we can observe with our five senses.

Of course, many items in our models are not directly observable but they create some observable effect. We have no place in our models for capricious or arbitrary entities. We don't assume that God or some other personal force has a place in our models. When we say a device has a "gremlin" we are kidding as far as scientific endeavor is concerned. If we debug a computer program, we do it with the assumption that a rational, reproducible problem is involved.

This approach to the scientific endeavor is significantly different from the view of philosophers earlier in this century. One school of thought, the logical positivists, believed that all reality could be ascertained through empirical methods, that is, through the extension of our five senses. That view said if it wasn't observable it didn't exist. Most of us today are not at that point. We see a scientific model as true when it is useful for prediction. We find that it is not a means of determining "absolute truth" or some other such philosophical concept. We have no hesitancy to use conflicting models. The most common example is that we look at light as being made up of electromagnetic waves to explain defraction phenomena, or we look at it as being made up of particles called photons, to explain the photoelectric effect. These two models of light are mutually contradictory.

With this point of view, one approaches a medical

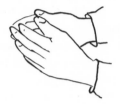

problem in terms of building a model for the illness and from that model predicting treatments. It is deliberately limited to what is physically observable. As a person of faith, I do not think that model can or has spoken one way or the other to the role of God or prayer.

A second perspective of mine involves the way God relates to the universe. I see God as overarching and totally pervasive. I see none of the limitations that we have as humans applying to God. We use anthropomorphic (humanlike) terms to describe God but these represent limitations in our ability to conceive of something, rather than an accurate description. It is not unlike our trying to describe in a scientific model an electron or quark or some other entity which we cannot know directly with our five senses.

I do not view God as a magic genie to call on when we are in trouble. I do not see God as working by arbitrary interventions into the scheme of things. Rather, I see a far more pervasive involvement in the design, operation, and working of the universe in which we find ourselves. That doesn't explain anything, but it says something about an orientation.

In the final analysis, I believe in prayer as an act of faith. I believe I am walking around today as an answer to prayers. How did God work? I think through the hands and minds of skilled physicians, through the effects of high energy radiation, through the physiological benefits of chemotherapy, through some endocrine flow as the result of positive attitudes, through the positive support from many friends, and through the gifts of a lot of individuals to a hospital drive before I came to town. There must have been other significant factors as well. Healing is too complex to be totally explained by any listing of factors.

The prayers that were offered for me by the pastor of the Goleta Presbyterian Church which we were attending were especially meaningful. Even though we had only started going to the church a few weeks before I became disabled, Don Hawthorne, the pastor, began calling on me regularly when I was confined to my home. As one would expect during a pastoral visit, he asked on the first occasion if I would like for him to pray for me. There were some little clues about the way he went about it that made his prayers special.

Having been active most of my life in a church, and having been involved many times with people who were praying for the needs of others, I have frequently been bothered by the attitude of some of those prayers. Often people pray, using the phrase "if it be according to God's will. . . ." That has often struck me as a cheap way out. It is sort of a no-risk way to pray. If the prayer is answered, one can say, "Great, it was an answer to prayer." If the object of the prayers is not achieved, then one can say that it was not "according to God's will."

I am fully aware of the Scripture in 1 John assuring us that if we ask according to God's will we will be heard. When I examine the context and the meaning of that passage, I do not believe it is talking about every little detail of our lives as being God's will or not. I think the context is a much larger scenario. When God's will is discussed in this context, I believe it means the broader sense of asking for things that are part of the whole scene of justice, understanding, and righteousness. It means not asking for things for the sake of making our life easier, better than others, or to let us avoid our basic responsibilities.

I see God's will as a comprehensive attitude, not a cataloging of a lot of little decisions as being "in" or "out" of a preordained plan. We have been made creatures of choice and those choices are genuine. God will be as happy if I like blue as if I like yellow, if I spend my vacation at the seashore or in the mountains, or if I am a chemist or a farmer. God will not find it pleasing if I lack integrity, use other people, or seek my own good at the expense of others.

Don's prayers took me seriously. He asked my permission to pray for me. He shared with me what he was going to pray for. He explained an approach in which he depicted an image of the expected result. He expected me to regain the use of my feet, to be able to get out of the wheelchair, to go beyond the crutches and cane, and to walk normally. One day he shared with me a little drawing in which he depicted an image of that result and in which he saw the support of my many friends as the mechanism leading to that end. I remember distinctly the first Sunday that I went to church without crutches or a cane. As I walked down the center aisle to take communion, my eyes met Don's and we shared a moment of deep understanding.

I am not sure what to make of it, but it is interesting to me to observe that the therapy recommended by the Simontons and the approach to prayer represented by

Don Hawthorne both involved forming an image of the result expected. In the first case I, as the patient, concentrated on the image and had it clear in my mind. In the second case, not only I but another person praying for me had the same well-defined image.

I have found some other moments of deep meaning in the religious sense connected with my illness. There was the night when I recognized that my muscles were continuing to deteriorate and were not improving. That was before the cancer had been diagnosed. It seemed clear to me that I would not get better. I prayed with intense desire. I asked that I might have thirty more years of life. In process of that prayer I received an inner assurance that I would, in fact, be granted that request. It has been a part of my assumptions ever since. It has been central in my expectations.

Certainly in many cases our prayers are answered by the changes they cause in the one asking. When Dr. Edwards was explaining the details of my diagnosis, her tone and comments suggested my life would likely be shortened by the illness. With the experience I've just recounted fresh in my mind, I replied that I expected to live for thirty more years. She replied, "Well, you'd better change your expectations. . . . No, I guess you can set any goal you wish."

My response was that I believed I could and that as my physician it was her responsibility to figure out how to get thirty more years for me! She has been doing her part. My expression of an expectation to live is helping me do my part.

November 1, 1981, is another day that stands out in my mind. The week before, I was given a complete physical examination, including a lot of laboratory tests and a full body CAT scan. It was the first full physical I had received since we stopped chemotherapy. The results showed that my blood had returned to a normal analysis and no visible sign of cancer showed in the scan. More than that, my legs were getting stronger and some movement had returned to my feet. With the help of my braces I was walking well enough that many people who encountered me did not realize that I was wearing braces on my feet or not walking normally.

November 1 was a Sunday and I was sitting with the other members of the choir at the Goleta Presbyterian Church. The Old Testament Scripture was Psalm 116. The words leapt out at me: "I love the Lord, because he has heard my voice.... The snares of death encompassed me.... When I was brought low, he saved me.... Thou hast delivered my soul from death, my eyes from tears, my feet from stumbling. I walk before the Lord in the land of the living."

The choir sang that grand Mormon hymn, "Come, Come, Ye Saints." I suspect my voice stuck out above the rest of the choir because I literally shouted the line, "All is well, all is well." Probably few around me realized the depth of meaning that service had for me.

8

Donald

My memories of the first months of my dad's illness are not distinct or too specific. Deb and I seemed always to catch on to things pretty much after they happened. The details of the types of tests and therapy, the emotions and feelings Mom and Dad went through, weren't clear to us until months later when we saw them again. Short phone calls and letters weren't enough to convey all that was going on. With patience I followed summaries of the process, not being submersed in it day-to-day.

What did have immediate impact was our submersion in the community of support which permeates the Goshen College campus. This we experienced day-to-day. Dad wasn't in serious physical difficulty with only the immediate family pulling for him. We had the prayers of many, many friends. The prayers weren't just intangible, idle well-wishing. I've become convinced that they served an integral part in Dad's recovery. To believe this was no small thing or to be casually assumed.

My faith in God before Dad's illness was naturalistic. God's hands were tied to the order first created. I'm not so simplistic anymore. Seeing the concern of friends here and the very nature of Dad's recovery linked to nebulous things such as attitude and will, as much as to medicine, helped push me to the acceptance of such a factor as supernatural intervention. Many other experiences have brought me to that acceptance also, but Dad's recovery stands out.

In the end, it matters little if God went out of the way or not. I can show no proof, which is the way it has always been and should be. What I present before all is the product—the life and the improving health of my father. Whether God's order was sufficient to bring about recovery or whether something miraculous is involved, either way, good was done; something I'll give praises and thanksgiving for.

9

Judy

No one ever thought to photograph my father in the hospital, or while he was in the wheelchair, and so I have never seen him in those confined states. It's hard for me to believe that he was that sick at all. When I left my parents in the summer of 1979 to study in Spain, Dad was as healthy and active as ever.

By the time I returned the following June, he had passed from health to serious illness and was well on the road back to health again. The changes in him seemed small compared to what I had imagined. He walked with a limp, and his hair was thinning out. He no longer took showers, since he was still too unsteady; in the evenings we listened to him singing loud and bawdy songs from the bathtub. But he was working full days, and riding his bicycle the three miles to and from work just as he had done when I'd last seen him.

I felt as if I'd lost my father and found him again. I hadn't known the man described in the letters I received in Spain—sick and getting sicker. During February, when Dad's condition was deteriorating but had not yet been identified as cancer, an unreported postal strike prevented mail from reaching me. That was the most difficult time, when I knew only that numbness and paralysis were moving rapidly up his limbs, and that there was no treatment. The only news I received came through a transatlantic phone call from a friend.

Later, when the letters began coming again, even the news of the cancer diagnosis was not as frightening as no news had been. Dad sent me several cassette tapes in which he described his radiation therapy and his attitude toward the whole experience. Hearing his optimistic voice worked miracles of reassurance for me; Dad became familiar again.

Here are a few excerpts from the journal I kept in Spain:

January 20, 1980

Mom and Dad called just now. I must have talked to them for twenty minutes, but it felt like five. It seemed so normal to hear their voices. Dad said that his problem was diagnosed as the Guillan-Barre syndrome. That means that things *could* keep on getting worse and reach the point of paralysis in his legs and then arms and it could eventually cause problems in digestion and breathing so that Dad would have to live in an iron lung. I'm crying as I write this. Nothing so serious has ever happened to any of us before.

On the other hand, the symptoms could turn around and go away and not recur. So far that hasn't happened, though; Dad says the numbness and pain are still spreading. How terrifying to watch helplessly as your body becomes more and more incapacitated.

February 11, 1980

There's a sense of lost security eating at me with the knowledge of Dad's illness.... It takes him so far from the happy, athletic fellow I've always loved. I haven't heard from Sally, Don, or Deb for a coon's age. I feel so far from my family. But I'm the opposite of homesick—I'm overused to this place and can't remember home.

February 20, 1980

I dream every night about Daddy. Last night he walked up to me and greeted me with a hug, and scolded me for saying in my last letter that I was afraid he would never walk again. I didn't say that, but that is my fear.

Right now things are particularly difficult. It's very, very hard not to know how my father is. I haven't received mail for three weeks now, not even a birthday card. At least I got to talk to John on the phone on my birthday last week. He gave me the only news I've had of Dad since I talked to Mom and Dad on the phone at the end of last month. He says Dad is in a wheelchair. I feel like banging my head on a wall. If Mom and Dad don't have time to explain things to me, I can understand. But I still need to know what's happening. That's why I'm having a rough time lately. No mail and for all I know Dad is in an iron lung by now.

March 29, 1980

Mom and I talked for some twenty minutes on the phone this Wednesday. She told me about Dad's disintegrated vertebra and how they are waiting to learn what the cause is. Daddy feels reassured that he will be healed. He was given that reassurance Wednesday night a week ago, when he couldn't sleep and was praying. I've never heard him speak of supernatural experiences before, so it's pretty impressive to me . . . . I started to imagine how things would be from now on if what Dad has is a tumor or something fatal. Suddenly it occurred to me that my children might never know him. I hadn't thought of that before, and I couldn't keep back the tears when I did.

April 9, 1980

I received a tape today from Mom and Dad. News, finally. They found that the vertebra that is the cause of Dad's problems is malignant. So now they are zapping it with radiation. Dad says it's ironic since he's lectured so often about radiation. It appears that the malignant vertebra can be zapped away, and Dad's neurological problems may go away, too, at least to some extent. He hopes to walk by May 1. The problem now is locating the original source of the cancer. That means more tests.

It's weird, but I'm not having trouble believing all this,

65

at least not from this distance. I keep remembering the time when our whole family was driving to Virginia. Grandpa was very sick and we knew we were going for his funeral even though he hadn't died yet. When we stopped for supper, Dad called ahead to tell Grandma how close we were and to ask about Grandpa. I remember very clearly seeing Dad walk back to us. We were sitting on and in the car, with all the doors open, munching on fried chicken.

"Well," he said, "my dad died about an hour ago." We'd been expecting the news and nobody cried or anything. We just got back in the car and continued on our way. I remember wondering why you don't know when someone important to you dies. Nothing had been any different at the moment of my grandfather's death than any other moment of that day.

We talked about Grandpa as we drove along. I'm always going to remember the impression Daddy made on me with his peaceful acceptance of Grandpa's death. He spoke with love about his father and you knew things were as they should be: another man had lived a full life and passed on to the things that come after.

Now I hear that same peace in Daddy's voice as he describes for me the diagnosis of cancer and the problems surrounding it. His faith and his sense of humor are a much stronger message than that dreaded word "cancer." Mom says the doctors like him because he asks intelligent questions and isn't all unraveled by the fact that he's got cancer. He's making the radiation therapy people come up with a joke a day for him. Mom says they're hard put to do it, but Dad is making a competition out of it.

I find myself wishing that I could have cancer, too, so I could sit in the hospital with him and play cards all day and make jokes about radiation rays.

April 25, 1980

Earlier Adela was telling Flor in hushed tones about my father's illness. They were in the kitchen and thought I couldn't hear them. I think Adela is afraid it would hurt me to talk about it, but, if so, she is wrong. I am only too willing to talk about it.

10

When It's Fatal

But of the approximately twenty-five individuals who worked in my office, three of us have had cancer. All of us have returned to our normal work loads. I am aware of five cases of cancer in the last two years among people who attend the same church I do. Two of us have returned to our normal activities, but the other three have died. A little over a year ago Owen Johnson and I were chatting at church about our therapy, commiserating about the loss of hair, and being positive about the results. Now he is gone, and I must admit every time I see his wife I have the reaction of wondering why I have been spared and he wasn't.

In the Indiana community where I lived for over twenty years, a number of my friends became ill with cancer. Some of them have recovered, but Ernest Smucker, Sara Hertzler, and Alta Hertzler have not. In these cases, we had some of the same support group, and sometimes the same physicians attending us. We had many of the same friends praying for us, but the results were not always the same. Why?

I find it helpful to think of life in the human body as a

net. It is not a single chain which is destroyed by losing the weakest link. The mechanisms that sustain life are not only complex, they have many contingencies and redundancies. A stroke may destroy certain nerve fibers, but others may provide an alternate path to accomplish the same functions. It is like being sustained by a complex net with many cross-links and many strands of varying size. We can lose some strands and others take over the support, growing stronger to handle the new load. In another case damage is done to a main strand and all the smaller strands together cannot compensate for the loss of the added load.

We cannot generalize so easily from one illness to another or from the validity of the treatment in one case to all other cases. We can know that certain factors help strengthen the strands of our nets. Good exercise, good diet, good mental attitude, and a good support group not only help keep us healthy, but also help our bodies to heal when disease strikes. However, we must always recognize that even under optimum circumstances, the strands of our nets deteriorate with time.

Cancer may tear at any size strand in the net. It would appear that in my case the primary damage was done to a smaller strand where the body's resources or the chemotherapy was able to repair the net. The secondary site in a vertebra was a bigger strand—to follow the analogy further. As it began to tear it would probably have ripped other smaller strands and torn the net. The radiation helped repair the damage. In some of my friends' cases the damage was at too vital a part of the net, or too much damage was done for a repair to occur. What we know is that each of our nets is sustaining wear and damage. Eventually each of our nets will tear.

In the case of some of my friends where the cancer struck more vital strands in the net, chemotherapy and other treatment, support of friends, and positive attitudes helped extend their lives. Certainly the support and positive expectations made the remaining months of their lives more significant and rewarding. The fact that they did not recover is not a negative reflection on them nor their friends. At the same time it does not negate the hope and healing that comes from the treatments—physical, emotional, and spiritual—that are available to those of us that get cancer.

It is God's plan that we die! The only thing that is negotiable is when. All the people healed in the biblical accounts, including those healed by Christ have long since died.

It is helpful to view life from a larger perspective. Each of us has but a brief moment in the timetable of the universe. Whether we live to be 50 or 80 seems important to us at the time, but the difference is not very significant on the larger scale of things. The quality of our lives during our brief time is of far more importance. Although Hutschnecker in his book concludes that "we do not die until we will to," he goes on to suggest that we are not always able to control our desire by rational means. The Simontons report that some of their patients, whom they have helped to develop positive attitudes, are almost apologetic when they find they are dying. They feel as if they have let their counselors down.

For all of us there will come a time when we are ready to die. It is part of the normal plan. We do not need to live in fear of it coming too early.

11

Vignettes

There are so many things associated with an illness one remembers. Many of them are small and not in themselves significant. However, one finds that it is the little things that make life difficult and they become major foci of one's attention when they occur.

Braces

Soon after the paralysis became sufficiently advanced that I could not raise my feet, the doctor decided that I should wear braces to prevent me from stumbling when I moved about with a walker or on crutches. A plaster cast was made of my legs and plastic braces were molded to fit. They were a godsend and made it possible for me to walk again after the cancer was treated and the leg muscles began improving.

I soon discovered, however, that after walking a little way my toes would be quite sore. An examination pointed out that the braces were pushing the toes against the end of the shoes but with the impaired feeling I couldn't tell it until they had rubbed for some time. It only required buying shoes a half-size larger to solve the problem.

As I started walking farther, I found that the limitation to walking was the soreness that the straps of the braces made on my shins. I kept looking for something to distribute the pressure over the larger area.

One day I was in an athletic store and noticed the plastic shin guards that soccer players wear for protection. When a pair of those were placed on the straps, the distance that I could walk was at least tripled. Both of these were minor points, but they made a tremendous difference in my daily life by little changes.

Hair

Soon after beginning chemotherapy, I was sitting in the bathtub taking a shampoo. As I rubbed the shampoo onto my scalp. I came away with handfuls of hair. For the next few weeks that preoccupied my thinking. Would I lose all my hair, or was there some way I could keep it from coming out? If I quit washing my hair, would it not come out? The doctor assured me that washing it or not would make no difference. If it was going to come out, it would do so in any event. In my case I lost only about half of my hair. Then one day I noticed a small fuzzy growth. My missing hair had started to return!

Where all of the hair that had been lost had been gray, the new hair was growing back black. Today my hair is not nearly as white as it once was and I don't even use Grecian Formula!

12

Debora

For me one of the most memorable occasions connected with Dad's illness was the first time he moved a muscle in his foot after almost a year of stillness.

Our whole family was home for Christmas vacation (1980) so we took off for San Francisco for a couple of days. The night it happened we kids, and Mom, were sitting in our hotel room watching TV. Dad had gone into the bathroom to soak his feet in the tub—a nightly ritual.

We had been quietly engrossed by the TV for some ten to fifteen minutes when we heard Dad's voice faintly from the bathroom. "Mary," he said. "Mary, could you come here for a second?" They were words we had heard all through our childhood but they carried an added emotion with them this time. Underneath that steady voice one felt just a hint of suppressed excitement sneaking out.

Mom got up and went into the bathroom while the rest of us gazed on at the TV. . . . We waited, but no sounds came from the bathroom. A hint of a question began to form in my mind. I glanced at my brother and sisters. They glanced at me. Then, all at once, as if the starting gun had signaled the beginning of a race, we were up from our seats and sprinting for the bathroom.

There Dad sat, with Mom at his side, both of them watching his feet floating in the warm water. Silence reigned as we watched Dad move his toes with a small but definite movement.

We stood there, engulfed by silence, unable to find words to meet our emotions. I stepped forward to give Dad a hug and kiss. Tears began to form and the silence was broken.

Even now I cry when I think about that moment because the love inside of me is too great to contain.

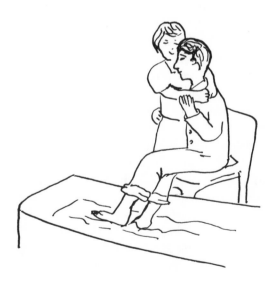

13

More Vignettes

Statistical Chances

Both Dr. Blum and Dr. Edwards were very helpful and continued to ask if I had any questions related to the illness or the treatment. Particularly when we were talking about the nature of the cancer, I felt that I was expected to ask the question about how long I might live. I never asked the question, and I really didn't want to know the answer, even if they felt they knew the statistical average for this type of cancer.

The reason I didn't ask has to do with my understanding of statistical data. Statistical data are useful when one is calculating the kind of treatment to give or evaluating the relative effectiveness of a given drug. I think it is not useful in an individual case. For example, the neurologist who examined me early in the illness indicated that there was a one percent chance that my problem could be caused by cancer. That is a chance of 1 in 100, but it was true in my case. Any individual case may fall within the upper and lower limits of a statistical range. If they told me that my life expectancy was six months or two years or five years, I would be tempted to plan and expect accordingly. I felt it was better to know that some cases are essentially cured and I would work on the hope and expectation that in my case this would be true.

In that vein, I remember distinctly the encouragement I received one day when Dr. Edwards told me that she had seen a patient with a condition similar to mine who had been free of symptoms for over seven years. I want to keep on thinking of myself as an individual and not a statistic.

Humor

I have found that people do not want to hear jokes about cancer. Of course, I may be jumping to that conclusion on the basis of too small a sample. I recognize that my family groans at what I consider to be my best efforts at puns in any case. But somehow I find that some sense of humor is necessary to survive a malady such as this. I thought I had a fairly respectable comment when I explained the neurological problem from the cancer by saying the "cancer had dropped to the limp mode."

There was one incident that occurred soon after I returned home from the hospital. I began awakening each morning with an extreme headache. I knew the doctors had been searching for the primary source of cancer and had not found it. Obviously headaches meant the brain was suspect. Then I remembered that they had performed a myelogram. In that procedure a dye is put into the spinal column and the patient is tilted under a fluoroscope to see whether or not there is any blockage in the spinal area. Usually after the procedure the dye is removed. In my case the vertebra was blocked at the damaged point and it would have left too small a volume of liquid if the dye had been removed, so they left it in. I am told it will slowly be removed over a ten-year period.

I recalled that the physician had said if the dye got into the cranial cavity it would not hurt anything but would give me a severe headache. Mary checked, and sure enough, my head was lower than the spinal column during the night because I was sleeping on my side. I started sleeping with two pillows and have not had a problem since. You can imagine my pride when I thought of two possible conclusions to the story. The first was that perhaps the myelogram explanation was correct, or maybe something had colored my thinking. The second was that maybe it was just the way the dye was cast. In any case, this may help explain why my family groans at times.

Rewards

Several of the authors I have referred to talk about noting the advantages of an illness. There are advantages. You receive a lot of attention. You take a vacation from work. You have time to read things you have been putting off. You discover both the number of your friends and the depth of their concern.

More than anything else, I believe a serious illness that threatens your life gives you a new perspective. Since I was sick I have had many conversations with friends who have also faced the possibility of death. Without exception our discussions and recounting of the experiences have had a level of understanding and a bond of shared danger that has meant a lot to me. In almost all cases we have talked about a new appreciation of life. We received a clearer picture of what is important. We have often reordered our priorities. It is true, all of us know life is finite on this planet. We know we have only a brief moment in the span of history, but at the same time we tend to put the thought out of our minds and live for the moment.

I am thankful for a new perspective—for a new appreciation of the world, for my friends, and for life itself. May we toast with Tevye in *Fiddler on the Roof,* "TO LIFE."

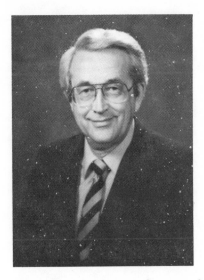

Henry D. Weaver is the deputy director of the Education Abroad Program of the University of California with headquarters in Santa Barbara, California.

He was born and grew up in the Shenandoah Valley of Virginia, but spent most of his professional life at Goshen College in Indiana where he was a chemistry professor and provost. There he was highly involved in the development of a study-service program which required Goshen students to spend an academic term abroad as a part of their general education.

He and his wife, Mary (Eby), have four children, all of whom were either in college or just out at the time of his illness reported in the book.

Weaver has a doctorate in physical chemistry from the University of Delaware and a bachelor's degree from George Washington University in Washington, D.C. He and his family have lived in Peru, Nepal, Poland, and Spain in connection with teaching or other educational assignments.